I0446571

THE HIDDEN DIARIES OF DOLORES CANNON: JOURNEYS AMONG LIVES

MEL DI BIASE

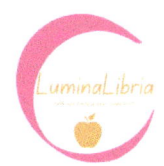

DEDICATION

To the reader,

This book is the result of passionate and courageous research that has delved into the mysteries of the soul and time. It's a journey among lives, showing us how we are all connected and how we can heal our wounds.

I invite you to read these pages with an open mind and a curious heart, allowing yourself to be guided by the voice of Mel di Biase, the author who has skillfully translated and interpreted Dolores Cannon's revelations.

I hope this book enriches and inspires you, just as it has done for me.

CONTENTS

INTRODUCTION

Alex's life, a psychology student with a restless spirit and a mind hungry for knowledge, had always been a tapestry woven with academic routines and philosophical inquiries. His world was a delicate balance between the tangible reality of university classrooms and the ethereal realm of psychological theories. But on a spring day when nature awoke with its colors and the sun's rays cast dancing shadows on the city streets, Alex's destiny took an unexpected turn. The discovery of Dolores Cannon's diaries in a dusty corner of an antique store was like the flutter of a butterfly's wings that would unleash a storm in his inner universe.

These diaries, bound in dark leather covers and marked by time, were like silent keepers of ancient secrets. Dolores Cannon, a name that resonated in psychology classrooms and the halls of soul exploration conferences, had been a pioneer, a traveler among the realms of the unconscious. In her diaries, Alex found not only detailed descriptions of past lives and stories of journeys through time but also accounts of encounters with mystical entities and phenomena that defied rational explanation.

With each page that Alex turned, he found himself immersed more deeply in a parallel universe of infinite possibilities. Dolores's stories were bridges connecting different eras, from ancient Viking warriors to noble Renaissance artists, each with their own story, dreams, and battles. These tales were open windows to worlds Alex had only dared to imagine, worlds that now seemed incredibly close, almost palpable.

But it wasn't just the stories of others that captured Alex's imagination. In the margins of the diaries, between the lines of Dolores's narratives, fragments of her personal life were hidden: her struggles, doubts, aspirations. These intimate revelations offered Alex a fuller view of the woman behind the words, a human portrait of an otherwise mythical figure.

As Alex delved deeper into the pages of the diaries, he began to perceive a mysterious connection between Dolores's stories and his own existence. Every experience of past lives, every encounter with the inexplicable, seemed to resonate within him with surprising familiarity. It was as if Dolores had charted a path that Alex was destined to follow, a path that would lead him to confront questions about the nature of the soul, time, and his own identity.

With a mix of excitement and apprehension, Alex continued his exploration of the diaries. He knew that every turned page brought him closer to a truth that could not only shake the foundations of his understanding of psychology but could also transform his entire perception of existence. It was as if he was traveling not only through the lives described in the diaries but also through the depths of his own being, on a journey that promised to be as exhilarating as it was unsettling.

And so, armed with an open mind and a courageous heart, Alex delved into the mysteries enclosed in the "Hidden Diaries of Dolores," ready to journey through lives, dreams, and realities in search of answers that could unveil the deepest secrets of the human soul and the universe itself.

EXTENDED PROLOGUE: ALEX, THE SOUL VOYAGER

In an old red-brick house, hidden among the winding streets of a city steeped in history and mystery, lived Alex. His room was a sanctuary, a corner of the world where time seemed to stand still, surrounded by towering stacks of psychology, philosophy, and classical literature books. Each book was an open window to a different universe, each page a step toward an inner journey that Alex undertook with almost mystical fervor. The walls were adorned with antique maps and portraits of psychologists and philosophers, silent guardians of his sanctuary of knowledge.

Alex had grown up in a family where a love for knowledge was a daily staple. His father, a university professor of history, had always encouraged his son to ask questions, seek answers, and never settle for the surface of things. Alex's mother, a librarian with a poetic soul, had nurtured his imagination with stories of ancient civilizations and epic tales. It was the evenings spent listening to his mother's stories under the starry sky in their small garden that ignited in Alex the flame of curiosity for the mysterious and the unknown.

In university, Alex distinguished himself with his acute

intelligence and his passion for psychology. But beyond textbooks and lectures, it was life itself that fascinated him: solitary coffee sipped while observing people, long nighttime walks through the city during which his thoughts intertwined with the hidden stories behind building facades and the fleeting glances of the people he encountered. Alex firmly believed that every person was a book to be read, an enigma to be solved, a journey to be embarked upon.

His thirst for knowledge often led him to places forgotten by most: dusty bookstores, historical archives, antique markets where objects from another time told silent stories. It was in one of these markets, in a secluded corner among shelves laden with memories, that his eyes fell upon Dolores Cannon's diaries. These volumes seemed to call to him, whispering promises of hidden secrets and journeys through time.

The diaries were like keys that unlocked doors to unknown worlds. As Alex flipped through them, an indescribable emotion welled up within him. Dolores's words, imprinted on those yellowed pages, spoke of past lives, journeys into the soul, encounters with the inexplicable. For Alex, this discovery was not just an academic enrichment; it was an invitation to a personal journey, a call to explore the deepest corners of the human psyche and perhaps, his own being.

Alex's dreams had always been vivid, almost real. In the wee hours, he found himself wandering through distant eras, conversing with historical figures, living lives that were not his own. These dreams, which some might dismiss as mere products of fantasy, were clues for Alex, pieces of a larger puzzle that connected to the stories in Dolores's diaries. Were these nocturnal visions echoes of past lives, or were they simply constructs of his knowledge-hungry mind?

His goal was not just to become a renowned psychologist. Alex aspired to unveil the deepest secrets of the human soul, to understand the invisible threads that connected past, present, and future, to explore the boundaries between science and mysticism. Dolores Cannon's diaries were the missing piece, the key that could unlock new horizons of understanding.

So, with a sense of discovery that transcended the academic realm, Alex began his journey into the "Hidden Diaries of Dolores." It was a journey that would take him far beyond the boundaries of his city and his life, an exploration that promised to reveal the most astonishing truths about human existence and perhaps, the very essence of time and reality.

HISTORICAL AND BIOGRAPHICAL CONTEXT OF DOLORES CANNON

In a humble house in a small town in Arkansas, nestled in a landscape where wheat fields stretched beneath an expansive and endless sky, Dolores Cannon was born. Hers was a family with deep roots, where the earth and the sky seemed to speak through the wind and the stars. In this corner of the world, where days flowed at the slow and reassuring pace of seasons, Dolores learned to cherish the simplicity of rural life, a heritage that would become the foundation of her existence.

Growing up in a time of transition, witnessing a world that balanced the solidity of traditions with the excitement of new discoveries, Dolores developed an early sense of wonder for the universe and its infinite possibilities. Young Dolores, with her curious eyes and a heart full of dreams, spent her days exploring nature, reading books that opened doors to distant and mysterious worlds, and listening to the stories of the town's elders, who recounted tales of bygone times and local legends.

Dolores's life took a decisive turn when, still young, she met the man who would become her husband. He was a Navy officer, a man with an adventurous spirit and an open mind, with an inexhaustible passion for hypnosis. At the time, hypnosis was viewed with some suspicion, an uncharted territory on the fringes of conventional science, a mystery that few dared to explore. Together, Dolores and her husband cautiously began to explore this field, driven by growing curiosity.

The early years of their research were primarily dedicated to hypnotherapy, using hypnosis as a tool to alleviate minor physical and psychological ailments. Dolores, with her innate empathy and sensitivity, proved to be a natural hypnotist. She started accompanying her husband in sessions, initially as an assistant, then as a full-fledged partner. Their home became a place of experimentation and discovery, where minds were opened, and the boundaries of reality were explored.

The pivotal breakthrough in their work occurred almost by chance during a hypnosis session that seemed like any other. A patient, immersed in a deep trance state, began to describe with astonishing detail a past life in a distant historical era. This unexpected event was like a spark that ignited an unquenchable fire of curiosity in Dolores. The doors to a new field of study opened before her: regression to past lives.

From that moment on, Dolores's work took a completely new direction. She began meticulously documenting every session, collecting stories of past lives that spanned centuries and cultures. With each story, with each journey through time, Dolores became increasingly convinced that she was touching something fundamental, something that could change the way we understand life, death, and the essence of human existence.

In the subsequent years of tireless research and practice, Dolores Cannon refined and perfected her revolutionary technique, which she named "Quantum Healing Hypnosis Technique" (QHHT). QHHT was much more than a simple regression methodology; it was a key that opened doors to unknown inner worlds, a bridge to memories buried deep in the subconscious. Dolores discovered that, through QHHT, her patients could immerse themselves in experiences of past lives with a level of detail and vividness that exceeded all expectations. These sessions were not just explorations of the past; they often offered new perspectives and solutions to current problems, providing patients with insights and healings that defied conventional explanations.

QHHT sessions became inexhaustible sources of fascinating narratives, and Dolores found herself navigating a sea of human stories spanning across centuries and cultures. She listened to tales of lost loves in forgotten times, battles fought in distant lands, ancient wisdom, and deeply human moments of joy and suffering. Each session was a journey into another life, an opportunity to better understand the human experience in its entirety. These narratives not only enriched the fabric of reality for those who lived them but also offered Dolores a broader view of human nature and the soul's journey through time.

However, Dolores's work transcended conventional past-life regression sessions. Her research led her to explore even more extraordinary and mysterious territories. Some of her patients, under deep hypnosis, began to describe encounters with extraterrestrial entities and experiences in other dimensions, advanced civilizations, and worlds far beyond earthly understanding. These accounts, pushing the boundaries of accepted reality, did not discourage Dolores. On the contrary, they spurred her to investigate further, to seek connections and meanings that extended beyond the limits of human knowledge.

The stories of encounters with other forms of life and journeys into alternative dimensions were imbued with messages and teachings that, according to Dolores, had the potential to transform human understanding of reality. The narratives often contained themes of cosmic unity, spiritual evolution, and an interconnection between all forms of life. Dolores began to see these accounts not only as isolated curiosities but as parts of a larger mosaic that spoke of a more complex and interconnected universe than could be imagined.

With a unique blend of courage and determination, Dolores Cannon continued her exploration of the most extraordinary and mysterious phenomena of human existence. Her work, documented in a series of books that encompassed a wide range of topics, became a source of admiration, debate, and inspiration for many. Through her publications, which included detailed transcripts of hypnosis sessions, personal reflections, and bold theories, Dolores initiated a new and stimulating dialogue between different disciplines—from science to philosophy, through spirituality.

Dolores's books were not just collections of intriguing stories; they were profound explorations of the human soul and its connection to the universe. On every page, Dolores sought to weave together the threads of these experiences, proposing theories about the evolution of the soul, karmic cycles, and the connection between different dimensions of existence. Her ideas, often on the edge of accepted reality and the realm of the possible, challenged readers to think beyond the limits of the known and to consider life from a broader, integrated perspective.

Dolores Cannon emerged as a key and pioneering figure in the field of exploring the human consciousness. By addressing controversial topics often avoided by mainstream science, she displayed an open mind and intellectual curiosity that led her to probe uncharted territories. Her work not only provided comfort and answers to those who participated in her hypnosis sessions but also inspired a global audience. Her unique approach compelled people to question the nature of existence, the reality of multiple lives, and the uncharted depths of the human soul.

Dolores Cannon's life was a journey of extraordinary discoveries, a path that transcended the boundaries of time and space, touching the remotest corners of existence. Through her research and teachings, Dolores not only contributed to the understanding of the human soul but also offered a guiding light to those seeking answers to life's big questions. Her legacy continues to influence spiritual and psychological research, providing a model for courageous and open exploration of the infinite possibilities of human beings.

In summary, Dolores Cannon's story is more than a tale of personal and professional discoveries; it is an invitation to look beyond appearances, to question the infinite possibilities of existence, and to embrace with courage the mysteries of the human soul. Her work and her life remain a tribute to her unwavering curiosity and her relentless pursuit of truth, inspiring generations to explore the depths of consciousness and being.

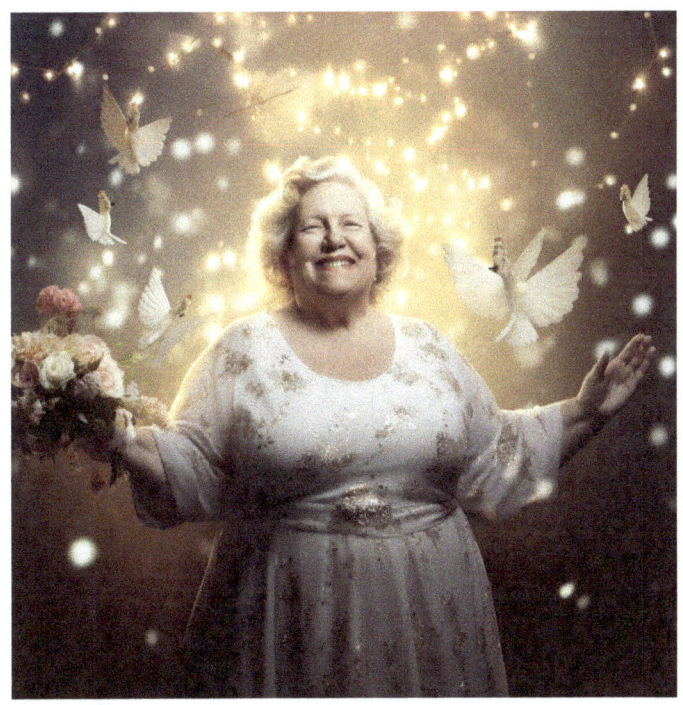

THE AWAKENING OF CURIOSITY

The Initial Discovery

On a crisp autumn afternoon, characterized by a clear and crystalline sky, Alex strolled down a seldom-traveled street in the city. It was that magical season when nature transforms, painting the world with warm and vibrant hues. The leaves, now weary of summer, had donned shades of gold, orange, and red, creating a soft and colorful carpet on the sidewalks. A light, fresh breeze gently wafted, causing the leaves to twirl in a silent dance. There was something in that autumnal air that spoke of change, mystery, and untold stories.

The street chosen by Alex was far from the hustle and bustle of the city center, a forgotten corner of the city where time seemed to flow more slowly. The streets were lined with small boutiques and antique shops, each with its dusty and enticingly mysterious windows. These shops were like guardians of hidden treasures, each with its own story to tell, each a small universe of memories and secrets.

Guided by curiosity and instinct, Alex found themselves in front of a particularly fascinating shop, almost hidden between the cream-colored facade of an old bookstore and the inviting aroma of a retro-style pastry shop. The shop, with its faded sign and creaky door, seemed to beckon. Inside, the atmosphere was thick with the past: a maze of antique objects, dusty books, and relics of bygone eras. Old clocks, black-and-white photographs, and vintage lamps hanging on the walls cast a soft and welcoming light.

Among the overcrowded shelves and showcases filled with curious objects, in a dimly lit corner almost forgotten by time, Alex spotted a wooden box. It was worn from use, with rounded edges and a patina of dust that told its story. Sealed and seemingly waiting for a long time, the box exuded an aura of mystery. With a heart pounding with excitement, Alex delicately opened it. Inside, hidden beneath layers of old fabric handkerchiefs, lay a series of ancient diaries, their leather covers darkened by time.

The moment Alex's fingers touched those covers, they felt a shiver run down their spine. It was as if they had touched a direct fragment of history, a portal to hidden and long-forgotten worlds. Their heart raced with a mixture of anticipation and excitement as they reverently flipped through the pages yellowed by the marks of time. Dolores's words, written in elegant and fluid handwriting, seemed to come to life, whispering stories of past lives, journeys through forgotten ages, and human experiences that transcended the boundaries of time and space.

In that silent shop, with the autumn light filtering through the dirty windows, creating dancing shadows on the walls, Alex immersed themselves in the stories told in the diaries. They felt the voices of people who had lived centuries ago, their joys and sorrows, dreams, and fears echoing within them. It was as if, at that moment, time had stood still, leaving them in a suspended limbo between past and present, in an intimate dialogue with the souls trapped within the pages of those diaries.

Alex found a refuge in the tranquility of the shop, a secluded corner where they could immerse themselves undisturbed in the reading. They settled into an old velvet armchair, once vivid in color but now faded by time, yet still warm and inviting. In the air hung a mixture of scents: ancient wood, yellowed paper, and a faint hint of old paint. It was an environment that breathed history, a perfect sanctuary for their new companions in their journey: Dolores Cannon's diaries.

The outside world dissolved like mist in the sun, leaving Alex on an island of suspended time. As they turned the pages, they felt transported beyond the boundaries of the present reality. The words in the diaries were like portals that led them to other eras, distant and forgotten places. Through Dolores's words, they lived the lives of people who had laughed, cried, dreamed, and struggled in remote times. Each story was a golden thread weaving into the grand tapestry of the human experience, each word a step in a journey through the depths of the soul.

Immersed in these stories, Alex began to sense a deeper connection with the fabric of existence. They realized that these diaries were not mere accounts of past lives; they were open windows to humanity, mirrors reflecting the myriad facets of human experience. In those pages, past, present, and future seemed to intertwine, revealing a universal truth that transcended time and space.

As the sun began its slow descent toward the horizon, shadows lengthened across the dusty shop window, dancing on the walls and creating a play of light and darkness. In that magical atmosphere, an insatiable curiosity began to sprout in Alex's heart. They understood that what they had discovered that day was much more than a mere academic curiosity; it was the beginning of a personal journey of exploration and understanding, a journey in search of answers to the great mysteries of human existence.

With Dolores Cannon's diaries held tightly in their hands, almost like a sacred treasure, Alex rose from the armchair. They felt that they had crossed paths with destiny, that they had opened a door to a new understanding of themselves and the world. With determined steps but a heart full of questions, they left the shop. Beyond the threshold, their journey into the mystery of human existence awaited them, a path guided by the thirst for knowledge and the desire to uncover the secrets hidden in the fabric of time and memory.

The First Journey

In the weeks following the discovery of Dolores Cannon's diaries, Alex's mind became a theater of endless questions and reflections. Every day, as they went about their daily activities, thoughts about the diaries besieged them like waves crashing against the shore. Curiosity and the desire to explore pushed them toward uncharted mental horizons. It was an almost palpable longing, a need for answers that led them to consider an experience of past-life regression, a practice they had only read about in Dolores's diaries.

Alex's decision to embark on this journey into the unknown led them to a small, simply furnished room, an oasis of peace nestled in a quiet corner of the city. The walls were painted a deep and tranquil blue, evocative of a cloudless night sky. A small window, adorned with a light linen curtain, overlooked a quiet garden where wildflowers danced under the afternoon sun's rays. The air in that room was filled with meditative serenity, isolated from the noise and frenzy of city life.

They settled into a plush armchair, its soft and welcoming fabric enveloping their body, conveying a sense of security and comfort. Their hands rested lightly on the chair's armrests, and their eyes slowly closed, following the gentle rhythm of their breath. The room was infused with a faint scent of incense, which seemed to accompany their thoughts on an inner journey.

The therapist's voice, calm and reassuring, floated in the air, guiding Alex through the levels of consciousness. Soft, rhythmic words invited them to let go, to travel beyond the boundaries of their conscious mind. The external world began to blur, like a painting losing its contours, and Alex felt themselves slipping into a state of deep trance.

In this state, time and space seemed to lose their usual meaning. Alex found themselves immersed in an alternate reality, a dimension where the past, present, and future interwove into a mosaic of experiences and sensations. It was as if they had opened a secret door within their soul, a door leading to reliving past lives, walking forgotten paths, and touching the very fabric of existence.

The sensation was extraordinary, almost supernatural. Alex felt every emotion, every thought of these other lives with a clarity and intensity that surprised them. Regression became a bridge connecting their soul to remote stories, allowing them to explore the memories and experiences of individuals who had lived in distant eras. This journey into the past was not just a discovery but also a deep connection with humanity across the centuries, a journey that would open new horizons in their understanding of existence.

As Alex delved deeper into the state of relaxation induced by regression, they began to perceive a subtle yet profound change in the atmosphere around them. It was as if the air itself had become charged with electricity, vibrating with unexplored possibilities. The boundaries between here and now blurred, giving way to a time-travel experience that exceeded every imagination.

Almost without realizing it, Alex found themselves catapulted into a radically different environment, a leap in time and space that left them breathless. It was as if a curtain had risen, revealing a world belonging to another era, a place steeped in history and mystery. They stood on a dusty road winding through an ancient village, a place that felt both foreign and surprisingly familiar at the same time.

The houses were sturdy stone constructions, with thatched roofs meticulously woven against an intense blue sky, a sky that seemed wider and closer than in their own time. The village was alive with sounds: the echo of people's voices conversing and laughing, the rhythmic clang of a blacksmith at work, the distant neighing of a horse. The air was filled with the earthy scent of the land and the sweet aroma of freshly cut hay. Every detail was so vivid and clear, every sound and smell so intensely real, that Alex felt as if they were truly there, a silent yet fully present observer in that bygone scene.

In their journey into this past life, Alex found themselves in the role of a young artisan, their hands marked by labor but their eyes lit with dreams and hopes. As they walked along the cobblestone streets of the village, every step, every movement was imbued with a sense of deep familiarity. They felt an intimate connection with the people they encountered, with their genuine smiles and curious glances. Conversations, even the most mundane ones, carried a deeper meaning, as if they were reliving moments from a forgotten life, rediscovering bonds and affections that had crossed the centuries.

Alex, in the body of this young artisan, felt the life of the village pulsating around them, a continuous flow of intertwined existences, a symphony of humanity lived in distant times. Every interaction, every exchange, every shared laughter seemed to weave a fabric of human connections that went beyond individual existence. It was as if, through this regression experience, they had opened a door to a hidden chapter of their soul, rediscovering a part of themselves that had always existed but had remained hidden deep within.

In the heart of that regression, Alex found themselves navigating an ocean of emotions, as vivid as they were varied. Each feeling was like a color on a canvas, painting the picture of a life lived with intensity and authenticity. Joy manifested in the little things: in the smile of a child running through the village streets, in the warm handshake of a friend, in the simple taste of freshly baked bread. These moments of everyday happiness shone like precious gems, illuminating the daily life with their light.

At the same time, the pain of losses made itself felt with a burning intensity. It was an ancient pain, a grief that resonated through the centuries, yet Alex felt it as if it were their own. The loss of a loved one, the separation from a friend, the fading of a dream: each sorrow carried with it a depth of feeling that Alex had never known before. And yet, amidst this pain, they also found a surprising strength, a sense of resilience that bound them to that past life in an indissoluble way.

The love for family and friends was a golden thread weaving through the experience of that life. Alex felt love in every hug, in every gaze exchanged by candlelight, in every comforting word in difficult times. It was a love that transcended time, a bond that extended beyond the boundaries of that single existence.

And then there was the fear of the unknown, a universal feeling that unites every human being. The fear of what cannot be seen or predicted, the tension toward the future. In that past life, Alex experienced this fear acutely, but also with a kind of quiet acceptance, as if it were part of the very fabric of existence.

When, finally, Alex emerged from the trance state, they felt as if they had been reborn. Regression had shattered the barriers of time and space, leading them to live an experience that defied all logic and rationality. They had lived the life of another person, yet that life had felt somehow intimately their own, as if they had rediscovered a hidden chapter of their own story.

Regression was not just a journey into a past life. It was the beginning of a journey of inner discovery, a path toward understanding the complexity of the human soul and its capacity to travel through time. Alex felt different, as if they had opened their eyes to a broader and deeper reality. That first regression experience had irrevocably changed their perception of reality and existence, marking the beginning of a journey of discovery that would take them far beyond the limits of the known.

TRAVELS THROUGH THE AGES

Multiple Experiences

After his first astonishing foray into the depths of past-life regression, Alex felt like a modern-day Marco Polo, a traveler at the edge of an uncharted new world. With each heartbeat, he felt an insatiable thirst for knowledge growing within him, a burning desire to further explore the annals of time and human existence. This newfound awareness became the compass that guided him on a series of extraordinary journeys through the ages, each unveiling fragments of past lives, weaving together a rich tapestry of human experiences.

In each regression session, Alex immersed himself in unfamiliar worlds, crossing the thresholds of distant civilizations. Each journey was a plunge into an ocean of culture and history, where historical details and cultural contexts were so vivid and profound that they surpassed all his previous knowledge. He found himself living the lives of people from different eras, each with their unique narratives, challenges, triumphs, and joys.

In one of these fascinating regressions, Alex found himself catapulted into the pulsating heart of an ancient Mesopotamian civilization. The streets were a maze of activity and colors, with bustling markets filled with traders, artisans, and farmers. He walked on dusty paths, flanked by imposing ziggurats that stood against a deep, almost ethereal blue sky. Majestic temples dominated the landscape, with their imposing sculpted facades narrating stories of gods and kings.

Alex, in the role of a young scribe, found himself immersed in a world where cuneiform writing was not only a means of communication but a sacred art, a bridge between the divine and the earthly. His fingers glided over clay tablets, tracing ancient symbols, words that were spells, contracts, and poems. He felt the weight of religious and social responsibility bearing down on his shoulders, a responsibility he carried with pride and humility.

Life in that time was a mosaic of experiences: daily rituals, moments of silent reflection under the starry sky, festivities in temples under the watchful eye of the deities. Alex, as a scribe, was a custodian of secrets and knowledge, participating in a world where the divine and the human intertwined in continuous dialogue.

The Mesopotamian world Alex experienced was rich with exotic scents - incense burning in temples, spices sold in markets, the aroma of bread baked in clay ovens. Sounds were a chorus of life: the clangor of the blacksmith, the chatter of vendors, the singing of priests during rituals. Every sensation was a thread connecting him to that distant life, every moment lived a step closer to understanding the intricate tapestry of human existence.

This regression was not just a window into a bygone era but a profound lesson in the continuity of human history and the persistence of the soul through the centuries. Upon returning to his own time, Alex felt enriched, as if he had lived a thousand lives in one, with each experience adding depth and meaning to his present existence.

In another astonishing journey back in time, Alex found himself on the wild and windy shores of a Viking land, a place where the sea and the sky embraced in an endless embrace. His hands, now those of a sturdy Viking warrior, gripped the oar of a long, slender drakkar, the typical Viking ship. His eyes, accustomed to mist and biting cold, scanned the misty horizon, looking for signs of new lands or imminent challenges. Under the gray and threatening sky, Alex, in that Viking life, experienced the impetuous desire for exploration and conquest, the thirst for adventures that defined his people.

But it was not just the craving for new horizons that defined that life. There were also strong family bonds, as strong as forged iron, and the importance of poetry and myths. Alex found himself sitting around crackling fires, where stories of gods and monsters, heroes, and legendary feats were narrated with a deep voice. It was a world where courage intertwined with destiny, where every action was infused with deeper meaning, woven into the intricate tapestries of Norse mythology.

In another regression, the environment changed radically, transporting Alex to the lush and sunny hills of Tuscany during the Renaissance. Here, he found himself in the role of a skilled artisan, his hands skillfully sculpting the cold, smooth marble, bringing statues to life that seemed to breathe and speak. In this life, every day was a tribute to beauty and creativity, a homage to the passion for art that ignited the hearts and minds of that era.

During that time, Alex, now a talented sculptor, was immersed in a world of intellectual and artistic fervor. Days were spent in the dust of his workshop, where marble took on divine forms under his expert hands, and evenings in the courts, where political intrigue blended with the fervor of artistic and philosophical discussions. It was an era where art was not just an expression of beauty but also a powerful tool for dialogue and power.

In this life, Alex experienced the complexity of human relationships within the Renaissance courts, where every gesture and word could have multiple meanings. He felt the thrill of seeing his works admired and discussed, the pleasure of contributing to the cultural ferment that would forever mark human history.

Each regression was a fascinating journey into a different era, a unique opportunity for Alex to personally experience the history, art, culture, and human relationships of distant times. These journeys were not just a series of historical experiences; they were deep dives into the soul of humanity, opportunities to understand the richness and diversity of human experience across time and space.

Every regression experience Alex lived was like a piece of a puzzle fitting perfectly into the vast mosaic of his existence. In these explorations of the past, he felt completely immersed in the lives of others, each emotion and experience lived with a completeness that transcended the limits of rationality. The pain and joy, the thoughtful decisions, and the moments of uncertainty of these people from the past resonated within him with deep emotional and spiritual resonance. It was as if, through these past lives, Alex was living a multitude of existences simultaneously, with each life adding a new hue to his understanding of the human soul.

These time travels not only greatly expanded his historical and cultural knowledge but also opened the doors to a universe of human experiences. Each regression was a plunge into a sea of emotions and perceptions, enriching Alex with a profound and transformative understanding. He began to perceive the delicate threads that connect all lives, a complex and intricate web of experiences, emotions, and wisdom that traversed time and space, weaving into a magnificent and incomprehensible design.

The regressions to past lives became for Alex much more than a series of journeys through history; they transformed into a profound exploration of the depths of the human soul. Each life he relived, each era he immersed himself in, each culture he explored added a new layer of understanding and empathy to his worldview. These diverse and varied experiences allowed him to tangibly grasp the complexity, beauty, and intricate interconnectedness of human existences, showing how each life, despite its uniqueness, is a chapter in a larger book, a note in a choir that resonates through the centuries.

Through these immersive and sometimes poignant experiences, Alex began to truly understand the fluid and interconnected nature of human life. Every laugh, every tear, every decision made by these souls from the past found an echo in his heart, teaching him that, despite the distances of time and space, there exists a common thread that binds all of humanity into a continuous and timeless fabric of existence and experience.

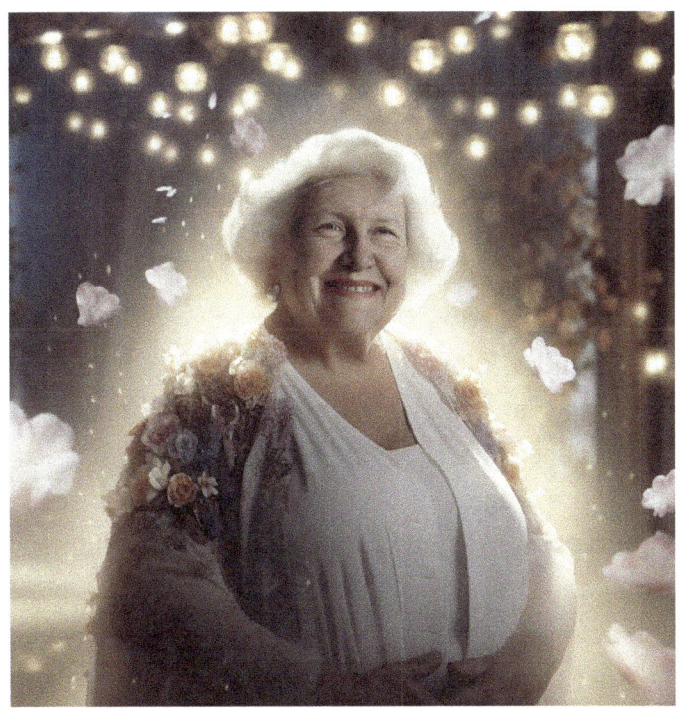

PHILOSOPHICAL REFLECTIONS

The numerous regressions to past lives conducted by Alex were not just journeys through epochs and cultures; they became sources of profound philosophical reflections. Immersed in this continuous flow of existences, Alex began to contemplate with greater intensity the universal themes of the nature of the soul, destiny, and reincarnation, themes that touched the deepest chords of his being.

The Nature of the Soul

As Alex delved into the depths of past lives, he was confronted with one of humanity's most enigmatic and ancient questions: what is the soul, really? Every experience lived during his regressions seemed to unveil a fragment of a larger enigma, a piece of a puzzle that extended beyond the boundaries of human intellect. These explorations led him to contemplate the soul not as a static singularity but rather as a river in perpetual motion, a dynamic flow of energy and consciousness.

In this view, the soul appeared as a living fabric, continuously evolving and transforming. Each past life that Alex relived was like a river flowing through ever-changing landscapes, shaping and molding the shores of his existence. These lives were not isolated from each other; rather, they were connected by an invisible thread, weaving together a narrative of growth and evolution.

Alex began to perceive the soul as an eternal traveler, a courageous explorer spanning epochs and cultures, living a myriad of experiences. In this cosmic journey, the soul encountered challenges and joys, pain and love, with each of these moments contributing to its growth and understanding. The soul, as Alex saw it, was a pilgrim on an endless quest for wisdom, meaningful experiences, and ultimately, an enlightenment that might reside beyond material understanding.

Past lives became metaphors for Alex's understanding of the soul's journey: each one represented a unique chapter in the grand book of existence, each with its own lessons to learn, obstacles to overcome, and moments of triumph. Through these explorations, the soul revealed its capacity to be resilient and adaptable, capable of rejoicing and suffering, loving and losing, always seeking new understanding, new truths.

In these deep meditations, Alex found a new perspective on the human soul. No longer an isolated entity or limited to a single existence, but a vital force on a continuous journey through time and space, a presence that transcended physical and temporal barriers, always seeking new experiences, new wisdom, a deeper connection with the essence of existence.

Destiny

Through his profound immersions into past lives, Alex began to contemplate destiny in an entirely new light. This exploration revealed to him that destiny was not a rigidly predefined path but rather a tapestry woven by human will, individual choices, and actions. Every life he relived in his regressions became a vivid testimony of how an individual's choices could shape not only their own life's course but also influence the destinies of those around them.

Alex began to see destiny as a complex and intricate dance between fate and free will. Each lived life was like a unique choreography in which individuals moved to the rhythm of their decisions, sometimes in harmony with the larger forces of the universe, other times in direct defiance of them. In this dance, destiny was revealed not as an unchangeable fate but as a field of infinite possibilities, an ever-changing landscape where each choice opened new roads and new realities.

In one of his past lives, for example, Alex found

himself in the role of a tribal leader, whose decisions not only determined the course of his life but also that of his people. Every choice, from the most mundane to the far-reaching, had the power to create waves of change. In another life, as a humble artisan, his daily decisions seemed of lesser significance, but over time, they proved to be fundamental threads in the tapestry of his community.

These experiences led Alex to a mature understanding of destiny. Every individual, in every life, was both the author and character of their own story, weaving the fabric of their destiny with choices and actions. In this view, destiny was not a static and predetermined path but a dynamic and evolving journey, where the freedom of choice intertwined with the mysterious and unfathomable forces of the universe.

The revelation of this complex interaction between free will and universal destiny became a source of deep reflection for Alex. He began to see life not as a series of random or predestined events but as a canvas on which each person painted their own destiny, a painting in constant becoming, where every brushstroke, every chosen color, contributed to defining the final design. This new understanding of destiny enriched Alex not only with greater awareness of his own life but also with profound empathy toward the lives of others, with each human being an artist of their own destiny.

Reincarnation

For Alex, reincarnation, once an abstract, intricate, and distant concept, transformed into a tangible and deeply lived reality. Every regression session became a journey through time, a poignant testimony of the soul's persistence across various bodies and eras. An entire universe unfolded for him where reincarnation was seen not as a simple cycle of birth and death but as an odyssey of learning and growth, a continuous process of soul evolution.

In each life he relived, Alex experienced a range of unique lessons, challenges to face, and triumphs to celebrate. These experiences led him to understand reincarnation as a journey of the soul, where each existence offered unique opportunities for learning, evolving, and maturing. Past lives were no longer just historical accounts; they were chapters in a larger book, narratives of a soul on an endless quest for wisdom, understanding, and spiritual growth.

Reincarnation, for Alex, revealed itself as an intricate interweaving of lives, each connected to the others in unexpected and surprising ways. He began to see how the actions, decisions, and experiences of one life could have repercussions in subsequent lives, as if each existence were a tile in a cosmic mosaic, contributing to the creation of a broader and more complex design.

These profound reflections on reincarnation led Alex to a deeper and more complex understanding of human existence. The nature of the soul, destiny, and the cycle of rebirth were no longer theoretical or philosophical concepts. They had become lived truths, tangible experiences resonating deep within his being. In this exploratory journey, Alex found not only answers to his questions but also found himself confronted with new questions, each answer opening the door to further mysteries and wonders of existence.

His exploration of past lives thus became an endless journey into the vastness of human consciousness, a journey that continued to unveil the hidden layers of the soul and being. Each regression was a step further in this journey, an adventure into the depths of the soul that revealed its eternal nature and its incredible capacity for transformation and rebirth.

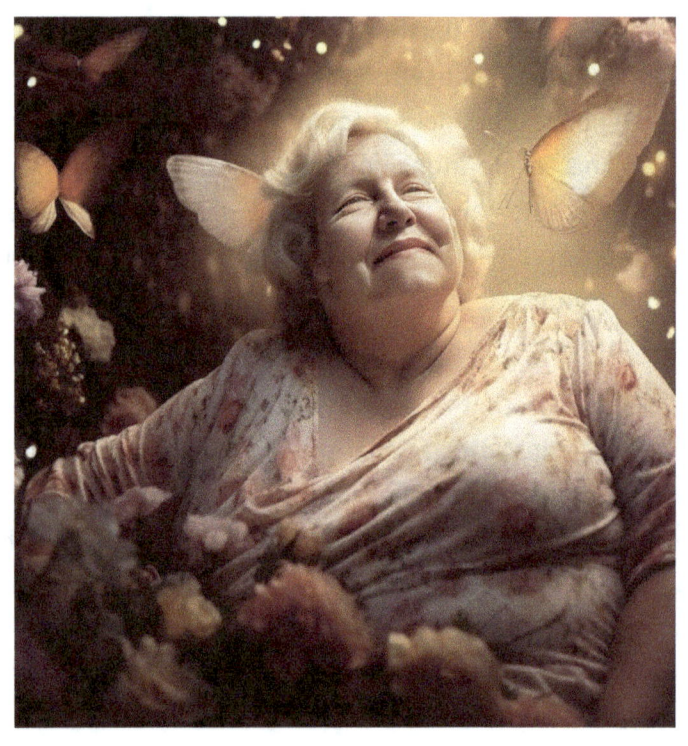

THE STORY OF DOLORES

Life and Work of Dolores

In his journey of exploring past lives, Alex became truly and deeply fascinated by the figure of Dolores Cannon. It was as if every page of her diaries and every word of her publications led him into a labyrinth of discoveries and revelations. As he read, he felt like he was unraveling the thread of a complex and captivating narrative, a path that brought him closer and closer to understanding the profound truths contained in the work of this extraordinary woman.

Dolores, born in a small town nestled in the countryside, grew up in an environment where simplicity intertwined with the richness of traditions and legends. Her childhood was marked by moments spent listening with dreamy eyes to the stories told by the village elders, stories that spoke of ancient times, heroes, and timeless mysteries. These tales fueled in her an insatiable curiosity and a deep love for the mysterious and the unknown.

From a young age, Dolores showed an innate inclination for knowledge and research. Her hours spent in solitude, with her nose in books and stories, forged in her a reflective and intuitive character. This love for stories, combined with a strong desire to discover and understand the mysteries of life, guided her along a path that would leave an indelible mark on the history of research into the human mind and past lives.

Dolores spent her youth in a constant quest for knowledge, exploring various fields of study, but it was her intrinsic attraction to mystery and the esoteric that eventually led her to work with past life regression. Her passion for storytelling and narration found a new expression in this field, where she could explore the deepest and hidden stories of the human soul.

As Alex delved into the life and works of Dolores, he discovered fascinating anecdotes and stories that spoke of her tenacity, limitless curiosity, and ability to connect with people on a profound level. He found out how, through her regression sessions, Dolores had been able to touch countless lives, offering comfort, insight, and healing to many.

Dolores Cannon, with her life dedicated to research and discovery, became for Alex not only a subject of study but also a source of inspiration. Her story was a powerful call to the power of curiosity, the pursuit of truth, and the importance of following one's passion, whatever it may be. Through his exploration of Dolores's life and work, Alex found a new understanding of the depth of the human soul and the infinite capacity for growth and transformation in the human being.

Throughout her career, Dolores developed a unique regression technique that allowed her to guide her patients into deep trance states, unveiling memories of past lives. One of the most fascinating anecdotes that Alex discovered was the story of a woman who, under Dolores's hypnosis, vividly and detailedly recounted her life in an ancient kingdom forgotten by modern history. The information that emerged during that session was so precise and detailed that, once verified, it left historians astonished, confirming the truth of those distant memories. This case not only strengthened Dolores's technique's credibility but also opened new perspectives on the hidden potential of human memory.

In another emblematic case, Dolores worked with a man who, during a regression session, revealed detailed knowledge of an ancient extraterrestrial civilization. The descriptions provided were so precise and coherent that they challenged conventional logical explanations, suggesting that the human consciousness might have connections to realities beyond our known world. This particular case opened the door to endless questions about the nature of human existence and our possible relationship with civilizations beyond Earth.

However, Dolores's work went beyond hypnosis sessions. Devoting much of her life to research and writing, she published numerous books that became foundational texts in the field of past life regression. In these books, she shared not only detailed accounts of her sessions but also her personal reflections and theories on profound topics such as reincarnation, the nature of the soul, and connections between different dimensions of existence.

Alex was deeply impressed by the stories of how Dolores Cannon, through her regression sessions and research, had a transformative impact on the lives of many people. He read numerous accounts of individuals who, after participating in her sessions, found not only comfort and understanding but also a profound form of healing. These people, often plagued by unanswered questions or unresolved issues, found in their past life experiences unexpected keys to unlock hidden aspects of their psyche and to answer questions they had carried with them for years, if not decades.

Alex read of cases where Dolores's clients, through regression, were able to overcome inexplicable phobias, resolve internal conflicts, and even heal from chronic physical and emotional disorders. These stories were powerful testimonies to the human mind's ability to find healing and understanding in ways that conventional science was only beginning to comprehend.

Alex's immersion in the life and work of Dolores Cannon became an endless source of inspiration and deep admiration for him. He was particularly struck by how Dolores, with great determination and courage, had forged an unconventional path in the pursuit of truth. Despite initial challenges and skepticism, she had paved new roads in the exploration of the human consciousness, radically changing the lives of the people she worked with.

Alex saw in Dolores a shining example of how the passion for knowledge and an unrelenting quest for truth could lead to revolutionary discoveries. Her story was a call to dare, to explore, and to transcend the limits of the known. Dolores had shown that, with curiosity and an open mind, one could discover aspects of human existence that remained hidden beneath the surface of ordinary consciousness.

The life and work of Dolores Cannon became for Alex not only a subject of study but also a continuous source of inspiration. Her journey was a testament to the transformative power of inner exploration and the importance of following one's passion, regardless of the challenges and obstacles. Her legacy, as Alex came to understand, was an invitation to deepen our understanding of the human soul and to explore the mysteries of our existence with courage and openness.

Personal Side of Dolores

In his research, Alex delved into the depths of Dolores Cannon's personal life, seeking to discover the human being beyond the researcher's figure. He was fascinated by how moral dilemmas, professional challenges, and personal relationships had shaped her life and work, providing a unique glimpse into the character and motivations of this extraordinary woman.

Moral Dilemmas

In Dolores's career, one of the most significant moral dilemmas revolved around the delicacy and responsibility of guiding clients through their past life experiences. Alex discovered that Dolores often faced the difficult choice of how deep to delve into regression sessions, especially when memories that could be traumatic or disturbing for clients surfaced. This aspect of her work was not to be taken lightly, and Dolores approached it with great care, balancing the need to explore these experiences with the need to protect the emotional well-being of her patients.

For Dolores, the key was to maintain a balance between the pursuit of truth and respect for the individual. Despite being aware of the potential emotional impact of her revelations, she was guided by a deep sense of ethics and a belief in the healing and transformative power of regressions. Alex read about how Dolores addressed these dilemmas with a compassionate and reflective approach, always attentive to the reactions and needs of her clients.

In these discoveries, Alex began to understand the complexity of Dolores's work and the weight of the decisions she had to make regularly. These moral dilemmas were not simple theoretical questions but real challenges that Dolores faced every day, testifying to her integrity and deep commitment to her work and clients.

Her philosophy of balance and honesty, as Alex discovered, was not just a part of her professional approach but reflected a profound understanding of humanity and the responsibility she had towards people seeking her help. Dolores, in her pursuit of truth, never lost sight of the importance of empathy and care, elements that defined not only her professional practice but also her interaction with every person who crossed her path.

Professional Challenges

During her career, Dolores Cannon faced numerous professional challenges, particularly the difficulty of gaining acceptance for her theories and practices in the mainstream scientific and academic world. Alex discovered that, despite initial skepticism and criticism, Dolores remained steadfast in her principles, continuing her work with unwavering dedication and passion.

Her path was filled with obstacles: she often found herself confronted by the scientific and academic community, which tended to view her methods and conclusions with suspicion and sometimes open skepticism. However, Dolores did not be deterred. She showed extraordinary resilience, convinced of the validity and importance of her work. This determination stemmed from a deep belief that her discoveries held significant value, not only for understanding the human psyche but also for expanding knowledge about the potential of the mind and soul.

Her battles were not only for the legitimacy of her techniques but also for a broader acceptance of the idea that the human mind could access memories of past lives. This challenge, which questioned many established scientific and philosophical paradigms, required not only courage but also deep intellectual integrity.

Alex read about how, over time, Dolores's work began to gain recognition, albeit initially in small circles. Over the years, her approach to past life regression garnered increasing interest and respect, even from some professionals in the fields of psychology and spiritual research. Her ability to document and present her cases clearly and in detail contributed significantly to this shift in perception.

The story of Dolores's professional challenges was a source of profound inspiration for Alex. It showed him that a passion for truth and a commitment to research could ultimately overcome resistance and open new avenues of understanding. Dolores's perseverance and dedication to her work became, for Alex, a clear example of how loyalty to one's principles and tenacity can lead to significant changes, both in one's life and in the broader world.

Personal Relationships

Exploring the personal side of Dolores Cannon, Alex encountered the richness and complexity of her private life. Through Dolores's own words, from her writings, and from the testimonies of those who knew her, Alex discovered a woman whose personal relationships were as deep as her studies.

Family Ties

One of the most evident aspects was her strong bond with her family. Despite her intense career, Dolores always made an effort to maintain close relationships with her family members, finding in them not only support but also an endless source of inspiration and strength. Alex learned how her roles as a mother and grandmother were imbued with love, dedication, and wisdom, and how her experiences with her family often provided valuable insights for her research and writings.

Deep Friendships

Dolores was also known for her genuine and lasting friendships. Colleagues, collaborators, and even former clients became close friends over time, often bound by mutual understanding and deep respect. Her friendships were characterized by a quality of empathy and intimacy that reflected her welcoming personality and open spirit.

Client Relationships

Dolores's professional relationships with her clients were marked by the utmost respect and care. She treated every individual she worked with as unique, creating a safe and comfortable environment for them. This empathetic and compassionate approach was crucial in helping her clients navigate the potentially turbulent waters of their past life experiences. Many of her clients testified that working with Dolores had a profoundly positive impact on their lives, highlighting her ability not only as a therapist but also as a person with great humanity and understanding.

Through this exploration of Dolores's personal relationships, Alex could gain a more complete understanding of the woman behind the extraordinary career. He discovered that her life was a tapestry of meaningful relationships, shared moments, and experiences that enriched both her and those who were part of her life. Dolores's story thus became for Alex not only a source of professional knowledge but also a shining example of how human relationships can enrich and shape a person's life, providing a broader and richer context for understanding her work and its impact on the world.

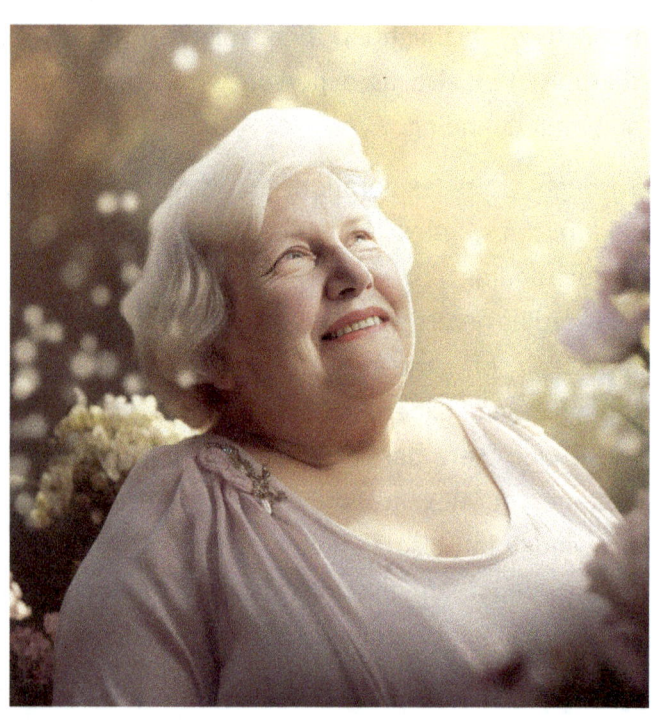

INTERWEAVINGS AND REVELATIONS

Surprising Connections

As Alex delved deeper into the world of Dolores Cannon, he found himself increasingly immersed in a narrative web that intertwined between his experiences of past lives and Dolores' own life. This network of surprising connections went beyond mere coincidence, suggesting a broader and more significant design.

One particularly fascinating element that emerged from his research was how the stories of past lives Alex had explored seemed to reflect, at times remarkably, the personal challenges, dilemmas, and triumphs of Dolores. These parallels were not merely anecdotal but deeply intertwined with universal themes such as the quest for truth, grappling with complex moral dilemmas, and the desire to connect with something greater than oneself – themes that had been central in Dolores' life and work.

In one of his most intense sessions, Alex relived the life of an ancient priestess, whose life path bore surprising similarities to Dolores'. Like Dolores, this priestess was a guardian of ancient knowledge, often misunderstood and occasionally isolated from her community. However, her dedication to knowledge and wisdom guided her, a direct parallel to Dolores' tireless commitment to her research.

In another regression, Alex found himself in the shoes of an inventor from a bygone era, whose innovative vision was initially met with resistance. This life reflected Dolores' persistence in pursuing her work on regression, despite initial resistance and difficulties. The story of this inventor, so similar to Dolores' tenacity, underscored the universal nature of the struggle against conventions to bring forth new truths.

These interweavings between past lives and Dolores' life not only enriched Alex's understanding of Dolores' work but also offered him a new perspective on the interconnected nature of human experiences. He began to grasp that every past life he had explored, every story he had relived, was not just a personal journey into the past but also a part of a larger narrative that intertwined with the lives of other people, including Dolores.

This revelation opened up a new dimension of understanding for Alex. He started to see Dolores' work not only as a collection of research and regression sessions but as a vital part of a universal mosaic of human stories. Each life, each experience, became a thread in a complex fabric that connected people through time and space, revealing a larger design in which Dolores' life was an essential element.

Alex began to perceive reality itself as an interweaving of multiple paths and stories, where connections and revelations continued to emerge in ever-new and surprising ways.

In a particular regression, for example, Alex found himself in the life of an ancient healer, whose challenges and successes surprisingly mirrored Dolores' career as a therapist and researcher. This character, like Dolores, had to face resistance and skepticism but remained true to their mission of helping and healing others. This discovery led Alex to reflect on how past life experiences could not only provide insight into an individual's personal history but also reveal broader connections and universal themes.

In one of his deepest and most transformative regression sessions, Alex found himself immersed in the life of a philosopher in an ancient civilization, an experience that resonated deeply with him, revealing striking parallels with the life and work of Dolores Cannon.

The Ancient Civilization

The philosopher lived in a distant era, in a civilization whose name had been lost to time but whose wisdom had left an indelible mark on human history. The society in which he lived was advanced and prosperous, with cities built of stone and marble, surrounded by lush gardens and aqueducts. It was a civilization that valued knowledge, art, and philosophy, and in which the philosopher found his true calling.

The Pursuit of Knowledge

The philosopher, a man of average height with piercing eyes and a long beard, spent his days in the city's library, surrounded by scrolls of parchment and ancient texts. He was known for his sharp mind and inquisitive spirit, always seeking answers to the great questions of existence. His thirst for knowledge was insatiable: he studied astronomy, mathematics, human nature, and metaphysics, trying to understand the mysteries of the universe and life itself.

Existential Questions

His research led him to contemplate deeply on the nature of existence and reality. He pondered the makeup of the universe, the meaning of life, and humanity's role in the grand scheme of things. These questions were not just intellectual exercises but deeply personal inquiries that touched the core of his existence. His philosophical inquiry was an inner journey as much as an exploration of the external world.

Parallel with Dolores

Reliving the life of this philosopher, Alex found striking parallels with Dolores Cannon and her work. Like the philosopher, Dolores had been a tireless researcher, an explorer of the depths of the human mind and soul. Their research, though separated by millennia, was united by a common desire to understand the inexplicable, to answer questions that went beyond the tangible and material.

The Impact of Regression

This regression experience left a profound mark on Alex. Reliving the life of a philosopher in an ancient civilization offered him a new perspective on his own quest for knowledge and understanding. It taught him that the pursuit of truth is a constant human endeavor, a thread that connects all epochs and cultures. This revelation not only deepened his understanding of Dolores' work but also provided him with a new view of his personal search for meaning and connection with the universe.

The series of interweavings and revelations that Alex

discovered during his past life regressions and his study of Dolores Cannon's work opened up a new dimension of understanding. He began to perceive Dolores' work not just as personal journeys into the past but as explorations of an immense and interconnected web of human stories, of which Dolores' revelations were an essential part. Each session, each discovery, each insight was a step closer to understanding this vast and complex design, a design that connected all human beings on a shared journey through time and space.

Connectivity of Experiences

Alex started to see Dolores' work as a bridge between the past and the present, between individual experiences and the universal themes of human existence. The regression sessions, which had once seemed isolated episodes, now appeared as chapters in a grand narrative that unfolded through time and space. This narrative was not just the story of specific individuals but also a narration of shared human experiences.

Dolores' Legacy

The depth of Dolores' research and her revelations about the mysteries of the human soul gained even greater significance in Alex's eyes. He began to understand that every discovery by Dolores, every insight gained from her sessions, contributed to a broader understanding of humanity and our place in the universe. Dolores' legacy, therefore, extended far beyond her writings and teachings; it was a vital part of humanity's ongoing journey toward self-understanding.

A Cosmic Design

Alex's newfound awareness suggested that every life and every experience was woven into a cosmic design, a tapestry that connected individual stories into a larger and more meaningful whole. In this design, Dolores' stories and her revelations played a crucial role, serving as links between different epochs and lives, and illuminating hidden aspects of human existence. This cosmic design went beyond immediate comprehension, suggesting that there are levels of connection and meaning that escape our daily perception.

Alex's understanding of Dolores' work and legacy became a fundamental part of his personal journey. He now saw his past life experiences not only as personal journeys into the past but as explorations of an immense and interconnected network of human stories, of which Dolores' revelations were an essential part. Each session, each discovery, each insight was a step closer to understanding

Union of Paths and Discoveries

As Alex's journey continued, his path and Dolores' discoveries seemed to merge, like two rivers meeting to form a single current. Dolores was no longer just a guide in the realm of past lives; she had become an integral part of Alex's personal story. Each new understanding of Dolores' research opened up new perspectives on his life, his relationships, and his purpose.

This personal revelation for Alex not only deepened his understanding of Dolores' work but also helped him see his own life in a new light. He began to perceive his own journey not just as a series of external events but as part of a broader inner path, intrinsically connected to Dolores' research and experiences. In Dolores, Alex found not only a source of knowledge and inspiration but also a spiritual ally in his personal discovery journey, one that continued to unveil the mysteries of existence and the deep connection between all souls.

Empathic Connection

In his journey through past lives and Dolores Cannon's work, Alex began to experience a deeper empathic connection with her. Every time he delved into regression sessions or lost himself among the pages of her writings, he found echoes of his own experiences and personal challenges. This process of introspection revealed an affinity with Dolores that went beyond a shared interest in regression and spiritual research. It was a connection that touched the deepest chords of his being, an emotional and spiritual bond that surprised him with its intensity and depth.

Dolores' words, the stories of her sessions, seemed to resonate particularly for Alex, as if they were written directly for him. He began to perceive that Dolores' discoveries and experiences were not just academic revelations but messages that touched universal themes of human existence—themes he grappled with in his personal life. Dolores' reflections on topics like the nature of the soul, destiny, and reincarnation resonated with the questions Alex had been asking himself for a lifetime. Each regression session no longer just offered a window into the past but also a lens through which Alex could better examine and understand himself.

This empathic connection allowed him to feel a sense of closeness with Dolores, almost as if her writings were personal dialogues with him. His research was no longer just an academic study but had become a personal journey of inner discovery, guided by the whispers of wisdom found in Dolores' experiences and words.

Through this empathic process, Alex began to see Dolores not only as a guide or teacher but as a kind of spiritual mentor, someone whose life and work mirrored and illuminated his personal path. Discovering past lives and Dolores' work became for him a bridge to a deeper understanding of himself, his personal challenges, and his spiritual journey.

Resonance of Stories

The stories that emerged from regression sessions and Dolores Cannon's discoveries began to resonate with Alex with a force and intensity that went beyond historical or anecdotal experience. He realized that his experiences of regression were much more than simple journeys through time; they were deep dives into universal themes that touch every human being. Love, loss, the search for meaning, and connection with the unknown—themes recurring in Dolores' work —began to find a deep echo in Alex's personal experiences.

As he progressed in his journey, Alex began to see his

regression sessions as mirrors that reflected not only past lives but also aspects of his deeper self. These themes, vivid in the stories told by Dolores, paralleled many of his internal questions, his reflections on his life's path, values, and existential purpose. Stories of love found and lost in past lives spoke to him about his own experiences of relationships and affections, while narratives of loss and overcoming helped him process his own griefs and challenges.

Furthermore, reflections on themes like the search for meaning and connection with the unknown offered him a new perspective on his spiritual and philosophical inquiries. The past lives explored were not just stories of others; they were also reflections on eternal themes of human existence, themes that Alex had always felt but not always deeply understood.

Each story, each relived experience in regression sessions, thus became an opportunity for Alex to explore and better understand himself. The connection with Dolores' stories became a powerful tool for self-discovery and personal growth. He began to recognize that through these stories, he could confront and resolve unresolved issues in his life, gaining a deeper understanding of his emotional and spiritual journey.

This resonance between past life stories and his

personal life led Alex to a deeper self-awareness and a more complete appreciation of the connection between individual experiences and the universal themes that define the human experience. Dolores' revelations, initially a means to explore the past, became for Alex a bridge to a more intimate and profound understanding of his present and life's journey.

Inner Journey

As Alex continued on his journey of exploring past lives and Dolores Cannon's work, his journey transformed into an increasingly deep emotional and introspective experience. Regression sessions and Dolores' books, once seen as windows into others' lives, began to reveal themselves as mirrors reflecting the hidden facets of his soul. Each story, each memory brought to light, became an opportunity for Alex to look deeper within himself, to explore and better understand his own emotions, fears, desires, and hopes.

This inner journey took various forms. In some regressions, Alex relived intense emotions that mirrored his deepest feelings—forgotten joys, suppressed pains, lost loves. These experiences helped him recognize and accept parts of himself he had overlooked or never truly understood. In others, through the stories narrated in Dolores' books, he found questions and answers that resonated with his personal existential inquiries.

As his journey continued, Alex realized that his regression sessions were not just forays into the past but also moments of deep reflection and personal growth. Dolores, with her work and words, had provided him with a key to unlock the doors of self-understanding. His explorations of past lives became a path to understanding how his past experiences had shaped his present, how every choice and feeling had contributed to the person he had become.

Alex began to see his research not only as an academic or spiritual path but as a journey of the soul. Each step of this journey offered him a clearer view of himself and the world around him. Through Dolores' discoveries, Alex found not only knowledge about past lives but also insights into his own inner nature and life's journey.

In this personal evolution, Dolores' figure became for Alex not only a guide in his past life research but also a role model and inspiration for his personal and spiritual growth. Dolores' understanding and wisdom found in her work became sources of inspiration and reflection, helping him navigate through the sometimes turbulent seas of his inner existence. His exploration of past lives transformed into a journey of personal and spiritual discovery, one that took him deeper into understanding who he was and who he wanted to become.

Union of Paths

In the course of his journey, Alex began to experience a union of paths with Dolores Cannon that went well beyond mere academic study or spiritual research. As he continued his explorations, Alex realized that Dolores' story and his personal experiences were weaving into a single, broad path of discovery. Dolores, for Alex, transformed from a researcher and guide to a spiritual companion, an entity that accompanied and guided him on his inner journey.

This merging of experiences and discoveries was not a random coincidence but rather a reflection of how Alex's individual path resonated with the universal themes addressed in Dolores' work. Dolores' revelations, which once seemed to belong to a distant and unknown realm, now became intimately linked to his own life, providing Alex with valuable insights not only into past lives but also into his personal path and spiritual quest.

This process of union of paths led Alex to a deeper understanding of himself and his place in the world.

He began to see the connection with Dolores not only as a source of knowledge but also as a symbol of his spiritual evolution. Each new understanding gained through regression sessions and reading Dolores' works became a piece that fit perfectly into the mosaic of his personal journey.

This deep connection between Alex and Dolores turned out to be a manifestation of the fact that every journey through life is inherently an inner journey. Every discovery, every experience, every encounter becomes an opportunity for introspection and personal growth. The bond with Dolores became a constant reminder for Alex that our external path is intrinsically linked to the inner journey toward self-understanding and one's role in the universe.

In this union of paths, Alex found not only a guide in his research on past lives but also a model and inspiration for his personal and spiritual growth. Dolores' story, with her discoveries and revelations, became for Alex a guiding light leading him to a deeper and more authentic understanding of his existence, illuminating the path to the heart of his true essence.

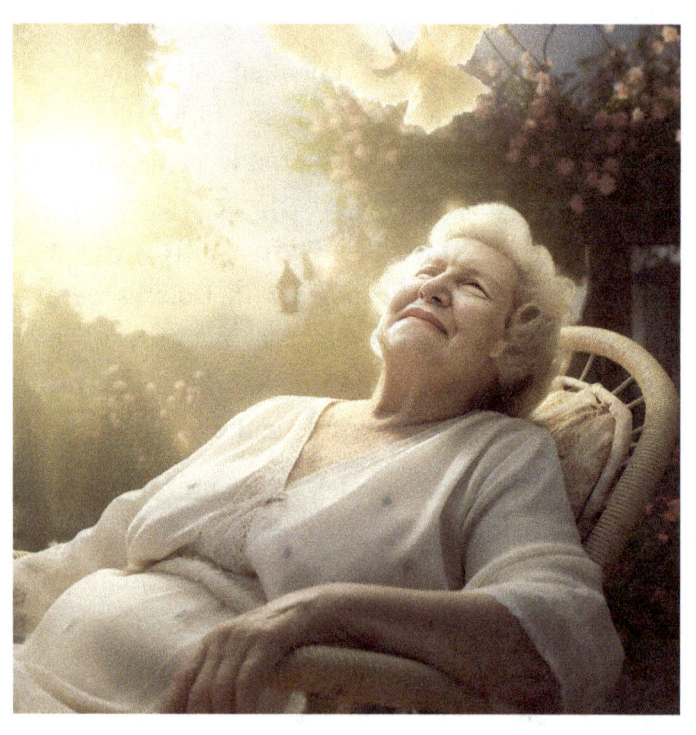

CONCLUSION AND REFLECTIONS

Climax and Revelation

As Alex approached the climax of his journey of discovery, he found himself facing a final revelation that had a revolutionary impact on his understanding of Dolores's work, past lives, and his own existence. This moment of climax was not just a revelation in the traditional sense but rather an enlightenment that carried with it a profound emotional and philosophical weight of enormous proportions.

The Unexpected Connection

In a particularly intense regression session, Alex found himself reliving a past life that not only had close ties to Dolores's teachings and research but also revealed an incredible personal connection to her. He discovered that he had shared a past life with Dolores, not as strangers but in a role that had a significant and direct impact on her life and work. This discovery was mind-boggling: Dolores and he had been, in some way, fellow travelers in a bygone era, bound by a destiny that transcended their current existence.

A Moment of Profound Revelation

This moment of revelation was accompanied by a wave of intense emotions for Alex. It was an experience that challenged all his expectations, offering him a new perspective on the intricate and mysterious nature of human connections across time. This understanding led him to contemplate concepts such as causality, destiny, and the interconnection of all lives. He began to see his journey not only as an individual path but as part of a larger design in which every life, every experience, is woven into a cosmic fabric of relationships and meanings.

Emotional and Philosophical Implications

For Alex, this final revelation had profound implications both emotionally and philosophically. Emotionally, he felt a sense of unity with Dolores that went beyond mere shared interests or academic discoveries. Philosophically, the discovery led him to contemplate deep truths about human relationships, time, and the very nature of existence. He began to consider the concept of souls reuniting across epochs, a theme he had always found fascinating in Dolores's research but now gained personal and direct resonance.

A New Vision of Life's Path

This revelation marked not only the end of his research journey but also opened the door to a new phase of understanding and personal growth. Alex found himself embarking on a new chapter of his life, one in which the lessons learned and discoveries made during his journey with Dolores became the foundation for a deeper exploration of his life's purpose and his role in the universe. Dolores's story and this incredible revelation became sources of inspiration and wisdom, marking a turning point in his personal and spiritual journey.

The Final Revelation

In his most transcendent regression session, Alex experienced something that surpassed all his previous encounters with past lives. Reliving this specific life was not just a journey through time but a genuine intertwining of destinies with Dolores Cannon. He discovered that in a past life, he had played a role as a mentor and spiritual guide to Dolores. He had been a figure of wisdom and enlightenment, playing a crucial role in shaping Dolores's early curiosities and interests in the mysterious and the unknown. This connection, extending beyond the bounds of time, had left an indelible mark on Dolores's life journey, paving the way for her future discoveries and research.

The emotional intensity of this revelation overwhelmed Alex. He not only felt surprise and disbelief but also a sense of interconnectedness and continuity that challenged his previous understanding of time and existence. His relationship with Dolores, now revealed, was much more than a mere coincidence of interests; it was a preordained bond, forged in another life and destined to unfold in this one.

This discovery led Alex to deeply reflect on the nature of destiny and the invisible tapestry that connects lives across time. He began to understand that his experiences of past lives were more than simple historical explorations; they were parts of a larger design, a cosmic plan that interwove souls in an ongoing dialogue between past, present, and future.

The final revelation was not just an endpoint but also a new beginning for Alex. He began to see his life and spiritual journey in an entirely new light, understanding that every encounter, every experience, had a deeper meaning and purpose. Dolores's story and this revealed connection became symbols of a much broader journey of the soul, one that continued to unveil the mysteries of existence and weave new threads into the fabric of his life.

Emotional and Philosophical Impact

The revelation of the profound bond between Alex and Dolores not only surprised him but also led him into uncharted emotional and philosophical territory. This discovery was like the last piece of a complex puzzle, suddenly offering him a complete and extraordinary view not only of his life but also of his place in the universe. The awareness of this predestined connection with Dolores prompted him to explore the depths of his soul, leading to profound philosophical reflections on destiny and the intrinsic connection between all human existences.

This moment of enlightenment brought forth in Alex a new understanding of the dynamics of life and the universe. He began to question the essence of destiny, wondering if human lives were guided by a preordained plan or the result of a series of random coincidences. The discovery of such an intimate and significant connection with Dolores compelled him to rethink concepts of causality and free will. He found himself reflecting on the idea that perhaps every choice and every experience were not mere isolated events but parts of a larger tapestry, woven into the fabric of existence.

The implication of this revelation was monumental. Alex began to see his existence not as a succession of arbitrary events but as a journey woven into a complex cosmic mosaic, where every soul, every life, is connected in ways that transcend human understanding. He started to perceive life as an interconnected flow of experiences, where every action, every decision, contributes to shaping the course of events in mysterious and intricate ways.

This new perspective led Alex to a profound realization: that every life is a thread in a universal fabric, intertwined with countless other lives in a design that goes beyond our immediate perception. His relationship with Dolores, far from being a mere coincidence or a chance encounter, was part of a larger cosmic plan, a dance of destiny that united their souls across centuries.

In this context, Alex found a new sense of peace and purpose. The revelation of his connection with Dolores not only opened new doors to understanding his past but also provided him with a compass for his future. With this newfound awareness, Alex looked to his future path with renewed curiosity and a desire to further explore the mysterious and meaningful connections that intertwine every life in an infinite dance of destiny.

Final Reflections

The final revelation did not mark the end of Alex's

journey but rather a threshold into a new era of understanding and awareness. This transformative experience opened his eyes to a vision of life that was much richer and more complex than he had ever imagined. Dolores's story, her research, and her revelations became for Alex not only sources of wisdom and inspiration but also a compass for navigating the sea of existence.

Alex's reflections on his past life experiences and his connection with Dolores led him to view his life as an ongoing journey of discovery and understanding. He began to perceive every event, every encounter, every choice as parts of a larger design, a work of art in life that was continually taking shape. The end of his journey with Dolores marked the beginning of a new phase in his life, a period of growth and deeper exploration of his inner self and the world around him.

With this newfound awareness, Alex approached the future with a renewed sense of purpose and curiosity. Every experience, every encounter, every decision gained new meaning and significance. He began to see himself not just as an individual on a personal journey but as part of a larger cosmic fabric, where every life is interconnected with countless others.

This new understanding led him to a more holistic and integrated approach to life. He began to evaluate his choices and actions not only based on their immediate consequences but also considering their impact on the broader fabric of existence. Dolores's story, with its revelations and lessons, became a constant guide on his journey, a reminder that in every moment of life, there is an opportunity to learn, to grow, and to connect with others in meaningful ways.

Ultimately, the conclusion of his journey with Dolores was not a conclusion but a passage into a new phase of his life, rich with potential and promise. Alex approached the future with a broader and deeper vision, eagerly ready to embrace new experiences and further explore the mysteries of the human soul and the universe. Every day, every moment became a precious part of an ongoing journey towards discovery, connection, and deeper understanding of existence.

EPILOGUE: ALEX'S FINAL REFLECTIONS

After embarking on a journey so rich in discoveries and connections, Alex found himself immersed in deep reflection about the meaning of his existence and his role in the universe. His interaction with Dolores Cannon and his experiences of past lives had transcended mere academic or spiritual research, triggering a series of profound transformations that touched every aspect of his life.

Personal Transformations

The most significant transformation for Alex was a profound reconsideration of his identity and his place in the world. His experiences of past lives, so intensely interconnected with Dolores's story, had greatly expanded his perception of reality. These journeys through time had challenged his previous beliefs about destiny, time, and space, introducing a new understanding of universal interconnectedness. He began to see himself not as an isolated individual but as an integral part of a vast and complex cosmic design, where every life, every choice, every moment held a meaning and impact beyond individual comprehension.

Connectivity and Unity

This new understanding led Alex to reflect on the connectivity and intrinsic unity of all forms of life. He began to perceive every encounter, every relationship as part of an intricate and meaningful network of interactions that defined the human experience. His relationship with Dolores, in particular, showed him how our lives can intertwine with those of others in ways that transcend linear concepts of time and space.

Reconceptualization of Time and Space

The discovery of his connection with Dolores in a past life made him reconsider the very concepts of time and space. He began to see the linearity of time as a limiting construct, realizing that past lives could subtly but significantly influence the present. This awareness allowed him to view his current life as part of a broader continuum, where past and future experiences intertwine and influence each other.

Reflections on Human Existence

These transformations led Alex to contemplate broader questions about human existence. He delved into the meaning of life, the role of the soul, and the evolutionary path of the human being. His exploration of past lives and his connection with Dolores had opened the door to a deeper understanding of consciousness evolution and humanity's search for meaning and purpose.

A New Perspective on the Future

With these profound transformations, Alex approached the future with a renewed vision. He felt a greater responsibility towards himself and the world around him, and a greater openness to continuous learning and growth. His experiences with Dolores had irreversibly transformed him, offering him a richer and more complex perspective on life and the universe. With this new awareness, Alex was ready to embrace his future journey with curiosity, hope, and deep gratitude for the countless lessons learned along the way.

Profound Realizations

In reflecting on his experiences and discoveries, Alex arrived at profound realizations about the nature of life and human relationships. He understood that his personal story was intertwined not only with Dolores's but also with the stories of countless other souls, each carrying unique wisdom and life lessons. This newfound awareness transformed the way Alex perceived every human interaction, seeing them not as mere chance encounters but as precious opportunities for learning, growth, and enriching his soul.

Interconnection with Others

This understanding led Alex to recognize and appreciate the deep interconnection between all people. He began to assess his daily relationships and encounters in a new light, viewing them as parts of a larger orchestra of shared experiences. Every conversation, every chance meeting, every friendship and conflict took on new significance, becoming moments of potential growth and learning.

Exchange of Experiences and Knowledge

Alex understood that life is a continuous exchange of experiences and knowledge, where every individual has something to teach and something to learn. Every person he encountered was seen as a potential teacher, a fellow traveler who, consciously or not, could offer valuable insights and teachings. This perspective made him more open and receptive in his interactions, actively seeking lessons and wisdom in every experience.

Enrichment of the Soul

The awareness that every interaction had the potential to enrich the soul transformed Alex into a seeker of wisdom in everyday life. He began to see every moment of his existence as an opportunity to expand his understanding of the world and strengthen his spirit. This led him to live with greater presence and awareness, recognizing that even the most challenging trials could be sources of enrichment and growth.

A Path of Continuous Growth

Finally, Alex came to realize that the journey of life is a path of continuous growth, an endless adventure where every experience, whether good or bad, contributes to the tapestry of our personal and collective story. Every person encountered, every experience lived was a piece that contributed to his personal development. With this understanding, Alex felt more connected to others and the universe, having discovered that true wisdom lies in embracing the journey of existence with curiosity, openness, and gratitude.

Application of Lessons in Everyday Life

Finally, Alex found himself applying the lessons learned in his everyday life. Every interaction, every decision, every new beginning was now seen as an opportunity to put the acquired wisdom into practice. This not only made him more aware and present in his relationships with others but also gave him the strength to face new challenges with a renewed sense of purpose and determination.

In this epilogue of his story, Alex found not only a deeper understanding of himself and his journey but also a clear direction for his future. Armed with the lessons of the past and inspired by the possibilities of the future, he was ready to embrace every new experience with curiosity, openness, and gratitude, continuing his journey of discovery and personal growth.

Renewed Sense of Purpose

The epilogue of Alex's journey marked a significant turning point in his life. Emerging from intense personal and spiritual exploration, he found himself endowed with a renewed sense of purpose and direction. The depth of his experiences, enriched by the connection with Dolores and the revelations about past lives, had triggered a radical transformation in him. Alex now felt a broader responsibility, not only towards himself but also towards the world around him.

This new understanding led him to live with greater awareness and intentionality. He was determined to make choices that not only fostered his personal growth but also positively contributed to the community. The realization of being so deeply connected to others gave him a sense of solidarity and commitment to the common good.

Inner Peace and Understanding

In his final reflections, Alex found an inner peace and understanding that had been elusive in the past. This peace did not stem from definitive answers or solutions to all the mysteries of life but rather from the acceptance of the journey itself as an essential part of human existence. He understood that every step of the way, every exploration, and every discovery were vital parts of a continuous learning process.

Openness to the Future and the Mysteries of Existence

Looking to the future, Alex felt excited about continuing his journey of discovery. Armed with renewed wisdom and a more open heart, he was ready to face new mysteries and explore the depths of existence further. He was determined to share the light of his discoveries with others, hoping to inspire and illuminate the lives of those he encountered.

Testimony to the Transformative Power of Inner Quest

Alex's story became a testimony to the transformative power of inner quest and the importance of every step in the journey of life. It demonstrated that the path of self-discovery is not only an individual journey but also a contribution to the collective fabric of humanity. Every discovery, every moment of awareness, every shared experience added to the ongoing development of the collective human experience.

In conclusion, Alex's journey became a symbol of humanity's relentless quest to understand itself and the universe. His story served as a reminder that, in the grand scheme of existence, every inquiry, every question, and every step forward have immeasurable value, contributing to the continuous evolution of human consciousness.

APPENDICES

To provide a more comprehensive understanding and enrich the context of Alex's journey, these appendices include historical, cultural, and academic insights. These notes and references offer additional readings, sources, and contexts that have informed and enriched his path of discovery.

Historical and Cultural Insights

Civilizations and Historical Episodes in Past Lives

Alex's past life regressions have taken him through a historical journey spanning various civilizations and crucial periods of human history. These insights provide a more detailed picture of these epochs, enriched by historical and archaeological sources.

1. **Ancient Mesopotamia**: Alex explored a life in this crucible of civilization, where the first city-states rose along the Tigris and Euphrates rivers. Details about cuneiform languages, ziggurats, and socio-cultural aspects of this era are provided, based on archaeological research and ancient texts.

2. **Viking Age**: Alex's life as a Viking warrior sheds light on Norse culture, navigation traditions, expeditions, and religious beliefs. References include historical essays and archaeological findings that illustrate the daily life and exploits of the Vikings.

3. **Italian Renaissance**: Reliving a life as a Renaissance artist, Alex experienced the cultural and artistic effervescence of 15th-century Italy. This section explores the historical context, artistic innovations, and social developments of this era, with references to artworks and historical documents.

4. **Ancient Extraterrestrial Civilization**: In one of his most unusual regressions, Alex explored a life in an extraterrestrial civilization. While this experience diverges from traditional historical narratives, speculative cultural context is provided, based on ancient cosmology theories and studies on the UFO phenomenon.

5. **Greek Philosophical Era**: Reliving a life as a philosopher in ancient Greece, Alex directly experienced the thinking and cultural context that laid the foundations of Western philosophy. References to classical philosophical texts are included,

contextualized within ancient Greek society and culture.

These historical and cultural insights offer a broader perspective on the past lives explored by Alex, allowing readers to delve deeper into the historical and cultural contexts of his regression experiences. Through these details, one can appreciate the richness and diversity of human civilizations and their influence on the course of history and cultural development.

Cultural Influences on Regression Practices

The practice of past life regression, as explored by Alex and Dolores Cannon, is not an isolated phenomenon but rather an activity deeply influenced by various cultural contexts and spiritual traditions. This section analyzes how different cultures and belief systems have influenced regression practices and the perception of past lives.

1. **Eastern Traditions**: In Eastern cultures, particularly in Hinduism and Buddhism, the concept of reincarnation is a fundamental component. These traditions have influenced the understanding and interpretation of past lives, emphasizing the idea of

karma and a continuous cycle of rebirth.

2. **Western Mysticism**: In Western mysticism, especially in esoteric traditions and New Age movements, past life regression is often seen as a way to access hidden wisdom and better understand one's spiritual path. These practices are influenced by a fusion of Eastern and Western philosophies.

3. **Transpersonal Psychology**: Within the field of transpersonal psychology, regression is considered a valuable therapeutic tool for exploring the subconscious and resolving traumas and deep-rooted issues from the past. This approach combines psychological methods with a holistic view of human existence.

4. **Indigenous and Shamanic Beliefs**: Many indigenous peoples and shamanic cultures practice forms of spiritual journeying that bear similarities to past life regression. These practices, which often include the use of rituals and trance states, explore connections with ancestors and past lives.

5. **Impact of Religion and Philosophy**: Various

religions and philosophies have different conceptions of the afterlife, the fate of the soul, and reincarnation. These ideas directly influence how people interpret and accept the concept of past lives and the practice of regression.

6. **Modern Adaptations and Developments**: In modern times, the practice of past life regression has undergone adaptations and developments, influenced by a growing fusion of spiritual and scientific ideas. This evolution reflects the increasing interest in the connection between science, spirituality, and understanding the human soul.

This section provides cultural and spiritual context that helps understand the variety of approaches and interpretations associated with past life regression, showing how these practices are a global phenomenon spanning multiple traditions and belief systems.

Academic and Scientific References

Dolores Cannon, known for her contributions in the field of past life regression and hypnosis, has written numerous books that delve deeply into these topics.

Here is a list of her major works, accompanied by a brief description of the key concepts addressed in each:

1. "**The Convoluted Universe**" Series: A series of books that explore complex concepts such as alternate dimensions, quantum physics theories, and unexplained phenomena. Cannon uses stories collected from her hypnosis sessions to discuss topics that challenge conventional understanding of reality.

2. "**Between Death and Life**": This book discusses experiences between death and reincarnation, based on testimonials from Cannon's clients. It explores themes such as the soul's process after death, past life review, and preparation for the next reincarnation.

3. "**Jesus and the Essenes**": Cannon explores the life of Jesus and the religious group known as the Essenes through regression sessions. The book provides an alternative historical and spiritual perspective on Jesus' teachings and his time.

4. "**Keepers of the Garden**": A book that explores the UFO phenomenon and the role of extraterrestrials in

Earth's history. Based on regressions of her clients, Cannon presents theories about extraterrestrial visitors and their influence on human civilization.

5. **"The Three Waves of Volunteers and the New Earth"**: In this book, Cannon discusses three different "waves" of souls that came to Earth to help the planet and humanity. It talks about how these soul "waves" are influencing change and spiritual evolution.

6. **"The Search for Hidden, Sacred Knowledge"**: An exploration of ancient knowledge and lost wisdom, delving into historical and spiritual mysteries through her clients' regressions.

Each of Dolores Cannon's books is based on hypnosis sessions with her clients and provides a unique exploration of mystical, historical, and spiritual topics. While her theories and conclusions have been a subject of debate and discussion, her works remain influential in the field of spiritual research and past life regression.

Recognized Researchers in the Field of Reincarnation and Past Life Regression

1. **Dr. Ian Stevenson**: Noted for his extensive work on reincarnation, particularly through research into cases of children who remember past lives. His works, such as "Twenty Cases Suggestive of Reincarnation," are considered foundational in the scientific study of past lives.

2. **Dr. Brian Weiss**: A psychiatrist and author of "Many Lives, Many Masters," Weiss is known for his approach to hypnotherapy regression, which he uses to explore the past lives of his patients. His books offer both clinical and anecdotal perspectives on past lives.

3. **Dr. Michael Newton**: Author of "Journey of Souls" and "Destiny of Souls," Newton explored the experiences of souls between lives through hypnotic regression. His works provide a unique perspective on the soul's progression and experiences in the afterlife.

4. **Journal of Regression Therapy**: Published by the International Association for Regression Research and Therapies, this journal includes research articles, case

studies, and theories in the field of regression and past life therapy.

5. **"Life Before Life: A Scientific Investigation of Children's Memories of Previous Lives**" by Jim B. Tucker: This book presents Tucker's research on children's memories of alleged past lives, providing a scientific analysis of the phenomenon.

6. "**Parapsychology: A Handbook for the 21st Century**" edited by Etzel Cardeña, John Palmer, and David Marcusson-Clavertz: This handbook provides a comprehensive overview of various aspects of parapsychology, including studies on past lives and reincarnation.

These authors and publications represent a significant part of research and academic thought on past lives and hypnotic regression. While some of these works tend to have a more open and speculative approach, others attempt to apply more rigorous scientific methods to the study of these phenomena.

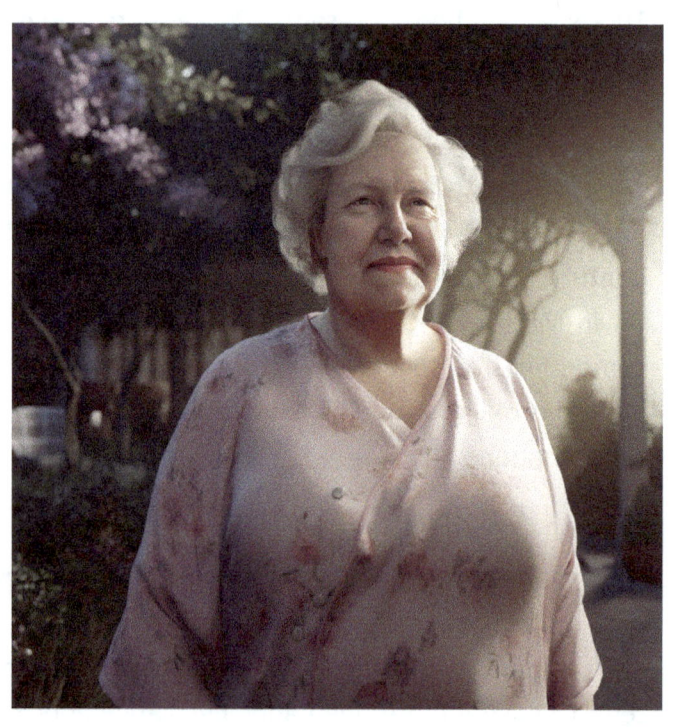

PHILOSOPHY AND PSYCHOLOGY: HOW THEY VIEW REINCARNATION, FATE, AND THE INTERCONNECTION BETWEEN LIVES

Philosophical and Psychological Theories on Destiny, Reincarnation, and the Interconnection of Lives

1. Eastern Philosophy on Reincarnation:

Hinduism: In Hinduism, the concept of Samsara describes the continuous cycle of birth, death, and rebirth. Karma, a law of cause and effect, determines the circumstances of each reincarnation.

Buddhism: Buddhism views reincarnation as a cycle of suffering (Samsara) that can be transcended through enlightenment. The concept of Anatta (no-self) challenges the idea of a permanent self that reincarnates.

2. Western Philosophy on Destiny and Free Will:

Stoicism: Stoic philosophers like Marcus Aurelius and Seneca saw destiny as a logical and inevitable order of the universe, with an emphasis on acceptance and individual virtue.

Existentialism: Philosophers like Jean-Paul Sartre and

Friedrich Nietzsche emphasize the concept of free will and personal responsibility in giving meaning to life.

3. Carl Jung's Analytical Psychology:

Collective Unconscious and Archetypes: Jung introduced the idea of the collective unconscious, a part of the psyche containing memories and shared ideas of all humanity, including concepts of rebirth and transcendence.

4. Daniel Dennett's Theory of Mind:

Materialism and Consciousness: Dennett, a philosopher of the mind, adopts a materialistic approach, explaining human consciousness and beliefs, including belief in reincarnation, through physical and biological processes.

5. Transpersonal Psychology:

Exploration of Altered States of Consciousness: This branch of psychology, with figures like Stanislav Grof, explores altered states of consciousness, mystical and spiritual experiences, contributing to a psychological understanding of reincarnation and the interconnection of lives.

6. **Philosophies of Death and the Afterlife:**

Platonism and Neoplatonism: These philosophical schools, based on Plato's ideas, often contemplate the soul, its immortality, and its journey after death, offering metaphysical views on successive lives.

7. **Philosophy of Consciousness:**

Contemporary Approaches: Contemporary philosophers like Thomas Nagel and David Chalmers explore the nature of consciousness, posing fundamental questions that can be connected to the understanding of past lives and reincarnation.

These various philosophical and psychological theories and approaches offer a wide range of explanations and interpretations of the themes of destiny, reincarnation, and the interconnection of lives, reflecting the diversity and complexity of human thought on these profound topics.

Alex's discoveries during his past life regression journey present significant psychological implications. Examining these findings through the prism of psychological theories can provide a deeper understanding of his experiences and internal changes.

1. **Freud's Unconscious Theory**: According to Sigmund Freud, the unconscious contains repressed memories and desires. Alex's past life experiences can be interpreted as symbolic manifestations of the unconscious, emerging during the hypnotic trance state.

2. **Jung and the Collective Unconscious**: Carl Jung proposed the concept of the collective unconscious, a reservoir of shared archetypes and symbols. Alex's discoveries can be seen as an exploration of this collective unconscious, where memories of past lives represent universal archetypes or common human experiences.

3. **Trauma Processing Theory**: Past life regression can be used as a tool to process and resolve past traumas. Alex's experiences might reflect a process of working through traumatic or emotionally significant events from his current or past life.

4. **Psychological Constructivism**: This approach suggests that our perceptions of reality are constructed by the mind. Alex's experiences during regressions could be interpreted as mental constructs that provide insight and personal understanding.

5. **Paul Ricoeur's Narrative Identity Theory**: Ricoeur argues that people construct their identity through narrative stories. Alex's past life regressions can be seen as an extension of this process, where he creates and integrates new stories into his personal identity.

6. **Transpersonal Psychology and Altered States of Consciousness**: Transpersonal psychology explores states of consciousness beyond the individual ego. Alex's experiences can be interpreted as transpersonal explorations that expand his perception of self and the world.

7. **Attachment Theory and Interpersonal Connections:** Alex's discoveries about his past relationships may reveal dynamic attachment patterns, influencing his current relationships and self-understanding in a social context.

8. **Kohut's Self Psychology**: Heinz Kohut's psychology of the self emphasizes the importance of relationships in self-formation. Alex's past life regressions can be viewed as a way to explore and integrate different aspects of his self, contributing to his personal development.

Through these psychological lenses, Alex's discoveries during his journey can be analyzed not only as metaphysical or spiritual phenomena but also as deep psychological processes that have had a significant impact on his identity, emotional well-being, and understanding of the world. This analysis offers a more comprehensive and multifaceted perspective on his experiences and transformations.

Personal and Social Impact

Effects of Regression on Personal Well-Being

Hypnotic regression, as experienced by Alex, has shown significant effects on the psychological and emotional well-being of individuals. These effects can be examined from various angles:

1. **Emotional Response and Catharsis**: Many find hypnotic regression to be a cathartic experience. During regression, individuals may relive and subsequently reprocess intense emotions associated with past events (real or perceived), which can be sources of stress or trauma. This process of emotional reprocessing can lead to a sense of release or resolution.

2. **Self Integration**: Regression can help individuals integrate aspects of themselves that may have been previously ignored or suppressed. This integration can promote greater self-understanding and self-esteem, contributing to a sense of completeness and personal coherence.

3. **Reflection and Personal Understanding**: Through regression, people often reach a new understanding of their current reactions and behaviors. Understanding the origin of certain behavioral or emotional patterns can be a fundamental step toward positive change.

4. **Impact on Mental Health**: Some studies suggest that hypnotic regression can have beneficial effects on mental health, including reducing symptoms of anxiety and depression. However, it's important to note that regression should be conducted by qualified professionals and is not a universal solution for all mental health issues.

5. **Spiritual and Personal Growth**: For many, regression offers an opportunity for spiritual growth. Exploring past lives or other transpersonal experiences can lead to greater self-awareness and a

renewed perspective on one's life and goals.

6. **Academic and Scientific Debate**: It's important to recognize that there is an ongoing debate in academic and scientific circles regarding the validity and effectiveness of hypnotic regression. While some studies show positive results, others question the truthfulness of recovered memories and suggest the need for further research.

7. **Controversies and Criticisms**: Hypnotic regression, especially when it involves past lives, remains a controversial topic. Critics question the authenticity of regressive experiences and caution against potential negative effects, such as the creation of false memories.

In summary, while hypnotic regression can have beneficial effects on the personal well-being of some individuals, it is essential to approach this practice with caution, awareness, and under the guidance of qualified professionals. Research continues to explore and better understand the breadth and depth of its effects on psychological and emotional well-being.

Contributions to Collective Understanding

The personal stories of individuals like Alex and Dolores Cannon can provide significant contributions to the collective understanding of humanity on profound themes such as spirituality, time, and existence. These contributions manifest in various ways:

1. **Broadening Perspectives on Spirituality**: Alex's experiences and Dolores Cannon's research offer unique perspectives on spirituality. They challenge and expand traditional understandings of concepts like the soul, reincarnation, and cosmic connection, encouraging a more open and inclusive dialogue on spiritual matters.

2. **Reconceptualizing Time and Existence**: Past life regressions and the theories presented by Dolores Cannon invite a reconsideration of conventional notions of linear time and singular existence. These narratives suggest that life can be understood as a continuum in which past, present, and future are interconnected and mutually influence human experience.

3. **Contribution to Transpersonal Psychology**: Stories like Alex's make significant contributions to transpersonal psychology, which explores aspects of the human psyche beyond the individual. These narratives support the idea that transpersonal experiences can have a profound impact on personal growth and self-understanding.

4. **Stimulating Research and Academic Debate**: Experiences of individuals like Alex and the work of Dolores Cannon stimulate further research and debates in fields such as psychology, philosophy, and theology. These accounts encourage academic exploration of concepts otherwise overlooked or considered marginal.

5. **Enrichment of Cultural Narrative**: Their stories add to the rich tapestry of human cultural narrative. By offering alternative and often innovative views on existence, they contribute to the diversity and depth of cultural discourse.

6. **Promotion of Empathy and Interpersonal Connection**: Listening to stories of past lives and spiritual experiences like those of Alex can promote a sense of empathy and connection among people.

These stories remind us that, despite superficial differences, there is a common core of human experiences and challenges.

7. **Influence on Personal and Collective Growth**: Stories of individuals like Alex and Dolores can inspire individuals in their personal and spiritual growth, encouraging a deeper exploration of the self and one's place in the universe. On a collective level, they can contribute to a shift in societal values and priorities, promoting greater spiritual awareness and interconnection.

In conclusion, the experiences and research of people like Alex and Dolores Cannon can significantly enrich the collective understanding of humanity, opening new horizons of thought and perception on the deepest questions of life. These appendices serve not only to provide a richer and more detailed context for Alex's story but also to encourage further research and exploration by readers interested in delving into these fascinating topics.

AUTHOR'S REFLECTIONS

In this personal section, I share my reflections on the connection I have developed with the subject of this book and my creative process during the writing.

Connection with the Subject

Writing Alex's story and exploring Dolores Cannon's ideas has been a profoundly personal and enriching journey for me. This path has allowed me to delve into complex themes such as spirituality, reincarnation, and human consciousness. I found a particularly strong connection with research on reincarnation and past lives, a topic that has always sparked my curiosity and interest in exploring the unknown.

Exploration of Profound Themes

As I wrote, I encountered existential questions that challenged me both intellectually and emotionally. Addressing themes such as fate and the interconnection of lives prompted reflection on the meaning of life and my personal understanding of the universe. I found that examining these issues through the lens of Alex's and Dolores's stories enriched my perspective and expanded my way of thinking.

Creative Process

My creative process for this book was characterized by a balance between rigorous research and free imagination. I was committed to maintaining the integrity and authenticity of the experiences described while leaving room for narrative creativity. This involved a careful navigation between accurate historical and cultural details and the creation of an engaging and inspiring story.

Challenges and Rewards

One of the greatest challenges was presenting complex ideas in a way that was accessible and engaging for readers. At the same time, it was incredibly rewarding to see how Alex's stories and Dolores Cannon's theories could weave together a narrative that I hope can touch, inspire, and perhaps even transform readers.

Personal Conclusion

In conclusion, writing this book has been a journey of personal discovery as much as it has been for Alex. It allowed me to explore the depths of the human psyche and reflect on the vastness of the human experience. I hope that readers can find in Alex's story a starting point for their own personal explorations and reflections, opening new horizons in understanding themselves and the universe that surrounds us.

NOTES ON THE GENRE OF THIS BOOK

The genre of this book can be defined as a hybrid of "spiritual narrative" and "metaphysical non-fiction." It combines elements of engaging storytelling with in-depth explorations of metaphysical and spiritual themes. The main features of the genre include:

1. **Spiritual Narrative**: Alex's story unfolds in a novelized manner, with a strong emphasis on his personal and spiritual journey. This narrative element offers readers an engaging and reflective story that explores deep existential questions.

2. **Metaphysical Non-Fiction**: The book also includes detailed analysis and discussions of concepts such as past lives, reincarnation, and spiritual connections, based on the work of Dolores Cannon and other relevant research. This non-fiction component provides a theoretical and academic context to Alex's

experiences.

3. **Exploration of Philosophical and Psychological Themes**: The book addresses philosophical and psychological issues concerning identity, time, consciousness, and fate, offering readers food for thought about the nature of human existence.

4. **Elements of Self-Help and Personal Growth:** Through Alex's journey, the book can also serve as a guide for readers in their personal exploration of spirituality and inner well-being.

In summary, the genre of this book sits at the intersection of spiritual narrative and metaphysical non-fiction, offering an immersive narrative that not only entertains but also stimulates reflection and personal growth.

AUTHOR'S NOTES

Mel Di Biase is an emerging author in the realm of spiritual and metaphysical literature, known for his innovative approach and the ability to skillfully intertwine storytelling with profound introspection. With a degree in psychology and a passion for both Eastern and Western philosophy, Mel has devoted much of his career to researching and studying the dynamics of the human soul and its infinite facets.

With a particular interest in past-life regression practices and theories of reincarnation, Mel has always sought to explore the boundaries between science, spirituality, and human nature. His debut book, "The Hidden Diaries of Dolores: Journeys Among Lives," is the result of years of research and personal reflection, representing a unique blend of lived experiences and academic knowledge.

Mel firmly believes that every individual can find a path of personal growth through understanding their past and present experiences. Through his writings, Mel aims to guide readers on a journey of inner discovery, offering them tools for a better understanding of themselves and the surrounding world.

When not immersed in writing or research, Mel enjoys

traveling, practicing meditation, and volunteering, firmly believing in the power of altruistic actions and the connection between all forms of life.

"The Hidden Diaries of Dolores Cannon: Journeys Among Lives" is just the beginning of Mel Di Biase's literary journey, promising to make an indelible mark in the field of spiritual and metaphysical literature.

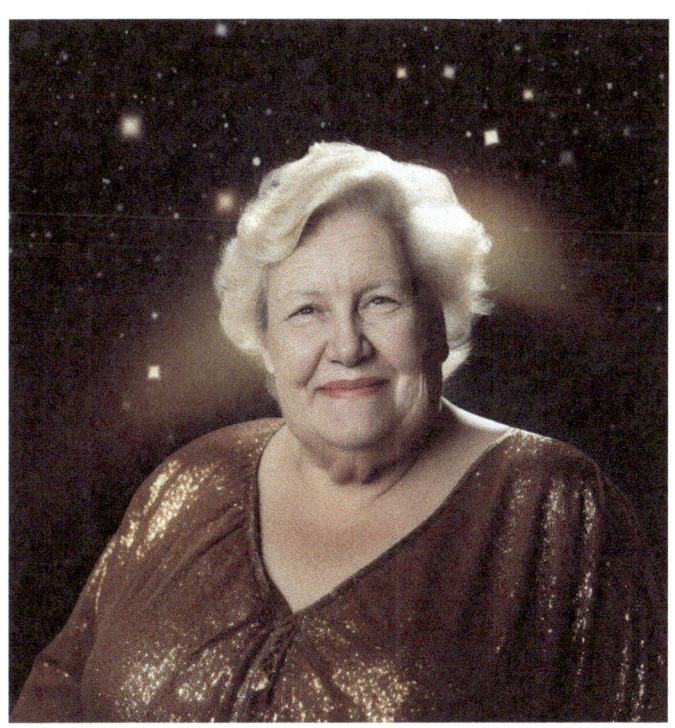

Discover a World of Knowledge and Inspiration

Visit www.libriutili.it

Dear reader,

We hope you have found inspiration and utility within the pages of this book. If your thirst for knowledge and personal growth is not yet satisfied, we have a special surprise for you!

We invite you to explore the world of LuminaLibria at www.libriutili.it, where a universe of books awaits you. LuminaLibria is an oasis for every type of reader, offering a wide range of genres to enrich your reading experience.

For Little Explorers: Browse our collection of Children's Books and Stories for Children, perfect for igniting the imagination and curiosity of the youngest readers.

For Art and Relaxation: Let yourself be captivated by our Coloring Books for Adults and Children, a creative way to relax and express yourself.

For Personal Growth: Explore our Self-Help, Personal Growth, and Biography Books to inspire and motivate you on your life journey.

For Curious Spirits: Deepen your spiritual journey with our Books on Spiritual Topics.

This is just a small part of what LuminaLibria has to offer. We believe that every book is a window to new worlds, ideas, and possibilities. Whether you're seeking adventure, knowledge, or inspiration, you'll find a book that speaks to your heart at www.libriutili.it.

Scan the QR Code below to begin your journey into the world of LuminaLibria's books.

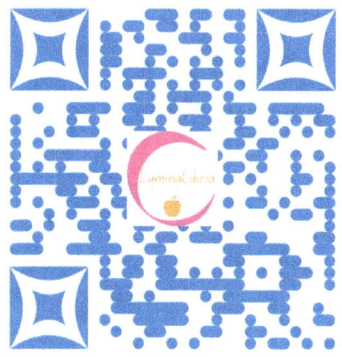

Thank you for accompanying us on this journey of discovery and growth. We are excited to see you explore even more with LuminaLibria.

Happy reading and continued exploration!

The LuminaLibria Team